KETO

Diet

THE COMPLETE GUIDE

First Published in 2017 by Oakleigh Publishing

ISBN-13:978-1974310968

Interior, Front and Back Cover Design by Oakleigh Publishing and Eva La Rouge.

Printed in the United States of America.

CONTENTS

AUTHOR

ACKNOWLEDGEMENT

INTRODUCTION

PART I

KETO CLARITY

PART III

KEEPING UP THE HARD WORK

AUTHOR

Eva La Rouge is a fitness coach, nutritionist, and grandmother to two beautiful grandchildren, and has struggled with her weight for years. After graduating from New York University with a degree in Health and Nutrition, Eva discovered the Keto diet back in 2008 and now enjoys renewed confidence, health, and well-being. When she's not busy looking after her two grandchildren, Eva works as a fitness coach at her local gym in Santa Monica, where she has helped thousands of women lose weight by following a Keto diet plan. She has especially taught her students how to successfully incorporate alcohol into their lives by discovering a 'must know' happy balance between drinking and dieting – the best of both worlds!

ACKNOWLEDGEMENT

"To my dearest Scott"

I would like to dedicate this book to my late husband Scott, without whom I would certainly not be the woman I am today. I'd like to say a big thank you to my doctor, Tim Renaldas. Without his advice, I probably wouldn't have started the Keto diet when I did. I'd also like to thank Sharon and Bill for all their support over the past 8 years. I'd like to give a shout out to Cindy from the WeightLossPro team, and Tom, Mike, Joshua, and the all folks from 101LifeHacks. Without their help and support, I wouldn't be the healthy, confident and happy woman I am today. Finally, I'd like to thank my two wonderful grandchildren for being a source of inspiration in my life. Kudos to all of you!

INTRODUCTION

I guess I won't be far wrong in my thinking that you've started, or are looking to start the Keto diet, and might be thinking 'can I drink alcohol on the Keto diet? If so, how much? What is the best kind of alcohol I can drink on this diet? Will drinking affect my weight loss goals? Will drinking ruin my Keto diet plan? If you've been asking yourself these questions, there is one thing I ask you to do right here and right now: STOP! Take a deep breath. Hold it. Now clear your mind of all the things you might have read on this matter.

Hi there! I'm Eva La Rouge. For the best part of 8 years, I have been on a Keto diet, and have been teaching it to friends, family and students from all around the world – students of different ages, sizes, sexes and background. From my humble beginnings in South Carolina, to my house here in bustling California, dieting has brought happiness to my life. Back in 2008, my friends, Bill and Sharon, spent a lot of time in and out of hospital. Sharon had lost her child at the time, and had gained a lot of weight comfort eating to cope with her loss. In a sense, who could blame her? Over the months, she gained a couple of dress sizes, and her weight was becoming more of an issue. After having a string of counseling sessions, she could cope better with her loss to such a degree that she now looked towards focusing on herself again. She was determined to be that slim, healthy girl she was back when she and Bill first met each other – and she achieved this. One year later, by sticking to the Keto diet, she was 70lbs lighter. Her confidence was through the roof. She now works as a weight loss coach at her local gym in Santa Monica. The rest is history! At the time, I was also suffering a weight problem of my own, but my problem was a bit different to hers. I'm a wine girl at heart. I love my wine! I'm what you would call a bit of a wine connoisseur at times. Diet after diet, the Atkins, Paleo and Zone etc., and year after year, I was not seeing the results I

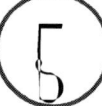

wanted to see. I questioned why I wasn't achieving the results my friends were enjoying. This suddenly changed when I watched the movie '⋯ First Do No Harm' starring Meryl Streep. In this movie, a young boy was treated for epilepsy by sticking to a ketogenic diet. A few weeks after watching this movie, I saw a couple of television advertisements talking about the benefits the Keto diet has for us ordinary folk. I thought 'That sure does sound good – almost too real to be true.' At my next doctor's appointment, I spoke to my doctor, Tim Renaldes, about starting the Keto diet. Although hesitate, he gave me the green light. After years of experimenting with a variety of different types of alcohol, it turns out, I was simply drinking too much of it! However, it was not the quantity of alcohol I was drinking that was the problem, but the type of alcohol instead. This is an importance distinction that I explain in this book. As I have come to understand over the years, not understanding this simple fact, does in 99% of cases, result in dieting failure.

This book

As we are aware, the marketing tactics behind modern weight loss are astounding. Expensive shakes and food products are sold to hopeful consumers all around the world, thinking that a flavor of the month solution will take care of their excess fat. However, as I have come to recognize over the years, the hard reality is that only a few weight loss methods work. The Keto diet, when executed in the right way, is one of these methods, and will not only help you lose a large amount of weight very quickly, but also improve your overall health and wellbeing.

Part I

To understand the Keto diet, we need to know how the body processes food. This involves a small history lesson - nothing too complicated! To keep it simple, it helps my students if they think of their body as a machine. Just like a car, we put in fuel and it travels from A to B effortlessly. At the pump, there are usually a few different options for gas, from regular to super – our body is much the same as this. Chapter one of this book 'The History of the Keto Diet' provides you with a brief, yet interesting story that traces how the diet has developed over the past 100 years. This may surprise you; it certainly did me!

You may have heard about the Keto diet being an extreme option for your weight loss goals. While many sceptics bleat on and on, saying that it is an unrealistic choice, largely because it involves almost completely cutting out carbohydrates, there are equal, if not greater numbers of academics and scientific evidence to support its benefits. One thing is for certain, for those of us who have tried it, these benefits are astounding, and I'm not just talking about weight loss. Chapter two of this book gets to grips on providing you with scientifically proven knowledge as to *WHY* the diet works – nothing too difficult!

In 2008, I was a much larger woman than I am today. After numerous trips to my doctor, having tried a plethora of prescription and herbal remedies, my weight loss wasn't improving. In fact, I was gaining weight. After starting the Keto diet, I didn't just benefit from weight loss (although that was the main intention of mine). I also benefited from profound spiritual, mental and personal changes that, through time, improved my confidence and overall well-being. I even had the renewed confidence to put myself out there in the dating scene! At the same time, however, it must be said that I did also experience a range of side effects in the first few weeks after starting the diet.

Part II

The basis of the ketogenic diet might seem quite strict to most people, and many people like to include alcohol in with their plan as well. You will discover how important it is to drink alcohol sparingly and choose drinks wisely according to carbohydrate content. The idea behind this is to maintain ketosis. We will discuss the pros and cons of including alcohol in your Keto diet plan.

Throughout the rest of the book, we will explore ways to incorporate alcohol into your daily meal plan in very small, but significant ways, with the goal of maximizing your weight loss and maintaining your confidence.

Next, we will move on to discussing the pros, as well as cons, of drinking on the Keto diet. More crucially, we will discuss how to maintain ketosis while drinking to help you to maximize your weight loss. We will discuss a range of alcohols. Those that are 'to drink', and those that are sadly 'not to drink'. We will talk about the nutritional content in this alcohol because this is the most important thing to consider when optimizing your Keto diet plan. Next, we will familiarize ourselves with guides for Wine, Beer and Mixed Alcohol. You will learn the things to look out for, and the things to avoid. Finally, we will celebrate ending this chapter with a list of the top 10 Keto friendly alcohols for your Keto diet plan.

Part III

In the final section of the book, we will talk about how you can maintain your dieting and drinking progress on the Keto diet. More specifically, we will introduce an optimized daily meal plan. This includes breakfast, snacks, dinner and, more importantly, which drink I feel is a perfect complement for your plan. If you have any unanswered questions by the time we get to the end of the book, there is a FAQs section that is a popular 'go to' guide for my students. You really should use this if you need to answer those burning questions. Finally, what better way to end this book than with a short quiz about the Keto diet. I hope you've been paying attention! Just kidding, the answers are also in there too!

Eva La Rouge.

PART I
KETO CLARITY

THE HISTORY OF THE KETO DIET

To get a handle on the Keto diet, I find that the best place to start is always at the beginning. In this case, history shows us that in the 1920s and 1930s, the Keto diet was used as a treatment for patients with epilepsy. This was the only help sufferers had until medications were developed in later years. An interesting fact is that, in 20% to 30% of all cases, the Keto diet remained more effective than medications in treating epilepsy. Today, despite our medical advancements, the diet is still used as an alternative remedy to treat it, as well as providing other health benefits discussed later in this book. In 1921, an endocrinologist by the name of Rollin Woodyatt, discovered that the diet helped our body in a remarkable way. It helped our liver produce three water-soluble compounds. These were β-hydroxybutyrate, acetoacetate and acetone. Together, these compounds are known as ketone bodies.

During the early 20th Century, an American by the name of Bernarr Macfadden, put forward the idea of fasting as a means of improving health. His student osteopath, Hugh Conklin, introduced fasting as a treatment method for controlling epilepsy. Coklin proposed that epileptic seizures were caused by a toxin secreted in the intestine and suggested that fasting for 18 to 25 days could cause the toxin to dissipate. His epileptic patients were put on a "water diet," which he reported cured 90% of children with the condition and 50% of adults. Analysis of the study that was performed later showed that, in fact, 20% of Coklin's patients became seizure-free, while 50% demonstrated some improvement. The fasting therapy was soon adopted as part of mainstream therapy for epilepsy and in 1916, Dr McMurray reported to the *New York Medical Journal* that he had successfully treated epileptic patients by prescribing a fast, followed by a diet free of starch and sugar since 1912.

Later, Russel Wilder, a medical student at the time, coined the phrase 'ketogenic diet' for its use in the treatment of epilepsy. After considerable research in the 1960s, scientists found that medium-chain triglycerides produce even more ketones per unit of energy. This led to a revised Keto diet for epilepsy sufferers that was drawn up by Peter Huttenlocher. Here, 60 percent of a patient's daily calorie intake now came in the form of MCT oil. This was a significant discovery because it meant that patients could eat more carbohydrates and proteins, which lead to the possibility of a varied diet. A larger variety of meals were now available for sufferers, and thus the Keto diet was born. And now we have the history behind the diet, let's take a look at it more closely.

THE SCIENCE OF THE KETO DIET

In a nutshell, the Keto diet is a low carbohydrate diet. The intention behind it is for your body to produce ketones as a source of energy. This happens when your body gets into a state called ketosis. This is achieved by eating fewer carbs (5% - 10%), more fat (60% - 75%) and moderate protein (15% - 30%).

What is ketosis?

Ketosis is the body's backup plan for when dietary fuel is not available. It pulls fat from storage and converts it to energy. Ketones are the by-products. Normally, our bodies process the carbohydrate we eat on an average balanced diet by turning it into glucose for energy. When ketosis is reached, our body begins to use the ketones produced from the transfer of fat to energy. If ketosis is maintained, our body can enter a metabolic state where it will continue to burn these ketones. Ketosis is not a foreign process for our body. It happens naturally when our glucose levels are low. As we have seen, this can help treat epilepsy, but can also help us optimize our weight loss goals, as well as improving our overall confidence and well-being. This process also helps improve our body's resistance to insulin, and so is often an excellent choice for diabetics – more of these benefits later in the book.

We mentioned ketones, but what exactly are they? When our body breaks down fat to use for energy, it produces certain byproducts. These are known as ketone bodies or ketones for short. The process works as follows:

- When our body doesn't have enough glucose, our glycogen levels will eventually run out.
- Our body now begins to burn fuel differently since the glycogen stores are now gone.

- It does this by using fat to fuel itself.
- Once the body uses fat for energy, which is known as beta-oxidation, our liver will start to produce ketones that fuel our entire system.
- When our body reaches this state, it is said to be in ketosis.
- This produces three types of ketone bodies produced:

  1. β-hydroxybutyrate
  2. acetoacetate
  3. acetone

Our metabolism is happy burning carbohydrates for fuel. Simple sugars from bread, rice, and sweets are broken down with little thought or energy, providing enough fuel to get through the day. If provided steady sources of carbohydrate throughout the day, things run smoothly. The problem is unless we are giving our bodies only what it needs for carbohydrates, the rest of those simple sugars will be stored as fat to use later, perhaps if you miss a meal. Weight gain happens when we consistently eat more than our bodies need to survive at any given time. Physiologically speaking, this is necessary so we don't keel over and die between meals, but these days, inactivity plus huge portions mean we will keep storing fuel we don't intend to burn – we gain weight.

When we do not have a source of steady carbohydrates during the day, our metabolism shifts to pull fat from our stores, and burn it for energy. This fat-burning process is called ketosis, and the byproduct of this is ketones. Ketosis is the body's natural back up to burning carbohydrates as a matter of survival. As you could imagine, ketosis helps us lose weight because we are constantly burning fat for fuel instead of burning carbs as they come into the system. The problem is, it takes a bit of time to enter ketosis, and as soon as we eat carbohydrates, the body goes back to burning sugars.

We can build our diets around proteins and fats instead of carbohydrates to mimic carbohydrate starvation to push our bodies into ketosis. While everyone will be a little bit different, the threshold of carbohydrates is about 50-60 grams per day, and about 10-15 grams per meal, before we exit ketosis. To put this into perspective, 15 grams is equal to a small slice of bread. To make the most of the meals, most of these carbs will be in sources like vegetables with low carb content. Check out the model meal plan in Part III of this book to jumpstart your diet.

The basic ketogenic meal is a combination of proteins like chicken and fish, with a large side of non-starchy vegetables like salad and zucchini. Fats can be used without real restriction as well, so healthy fats like olive oil and avocado can be used to make up for the calories not taken up by carbohydrate-rich starches like rice and potato. Here is a brief list of what is allowed on the Keto diet:

Proteins	Vegetables
Chicken	Lettuce
Fish	Tomato
Beef	Spinach

Pork	Green beans
Turkey	Zucchini
Eggs	Cabbage/Cole slaw

Overeating any of these vegetables could set you over your carbohydrate goal, so make sure to keep track of grams of carbohydrate per serving. Keep in mind that you can also have starchier vegetables like broccoli and carrots in smaller portions. Use online resources for lists of common food carb contents and apps like MyFitnessPal to track total carb intake.

If you have been a good guinea pig and following the rules, how do you know if you are in ketosis? Recent advances in science have developed test strips to test urine for ketones. A small number of ketones will be flushed out of the system in urine during ketosis, so if they are present in your urine, you are in ketosis. Testing regularly throughout the process can help you gauge just how high your carbohydrate tolerance is. The 50-60gram guideline is just that, a guideline. Some people will enter ketosis at higher or lower levels of carbs, making testing necessary.

Like any good diet, there must be some sort of calorie goal. Any type of food in excess will be stored as fat for later use. With the Keto diet, the food options are limited mainly to proteins and vegetables, which are naturally low calorie. It will likely be difficult to even max out your calories, but it is important to stay within a good range to maintain calories.

The average active person will need somewhere between 1600 and 2200 calories daily depending on age, sex current weight and activity level. It may feel like you are eating too much food, but vegetables are low calorie, so it is very easy to under eat on a Keto plan. Use the guide in part III of this book to help make your meal plan.

To determine your individual calorie needs, use a trusted online calculator or consult with a doctor or registered dietitian. The good news is, it takes a ton of non-starchy vegetables to exceed calories, so you will likely be overstuffed before that ever happens. If you can be disciplined enough to maintain ketosis for good stretches of time, the diet will help you lose weight. Most people fail in this discipline, adding in carbohydrates that quickly pull them back to burning them for fuel. Once ketosis is entered, the body doesn't really crave any carbohydrates, but getting over that hump can be difficult. Stick to your guns, get over carbohydrates and lose weight with ketosis.

HOW DOES THE KETO DIET COMPARE TO OTHER DIETS?

~CHAPTER 3~

Now that's an interesting question. Why? Well in some cases, the difference between certain diets and the Keto diet is as big as day and night. In other cases, there are diets fairly like it, but with minor differences here and there.

Let's look at a Keto diet again before we compare. The ratios of carbohydrates/fat/protein taken in daily are:

- Carbohydrates 5%-10%
- Fat 60% - 75%
- Protein 15% - 30%

Now let's compare this with other diets.

The Keto Diet Vs A Balanced Diet (from most nutritional experts):

Although a balanced diet might vary amongst nutritional experts, it is usually broken down as follows:

- Carbohydrates 45% to 65%
- Fat 20% to 35%
- Protein 10% to 30%

The Keto Diet Vs The Paleo diet:

With the Paleo diet, the ratio of carbohydrates, protein, and fat is as follows:

- Carbohydrates 22% to 40%
- Fat 28% to 47%
- Protein 19% to 35%

The Keto Diet Vs The Zone diet:

The popular Zone diet has the following macronutrient ratios:

- Carbohydrates 40%
- Fat 30%
- Protein 30%

The Keto Diet Vs The Atkins Diet:

When looking at the macronutrient ratios for the Atkins diet, you can see they are similar to those of the Keto diet.

- Carbohydrates 5%
- Fat 60%
- Protein 35%

THE BENEFITS OF THE KETO DIET

~CHAPTER 4~

Weight loss

Weight loss is arguably the most beneficial benefit of the Keto diet. When you reach a state of ketosis, your body burns fat to produce ketones. In many respects, your body is much like a machine. It burns fat in the most efficient way possible by tapping into your fat reserves all around your body – but cannot spot reduce!

Improved Mental Focus

As you progress further into the Keto diet, you might notice that you can concentrate and focus on tasks more effectively than you could before.

There is plenty of scientific evidence to suggest that. as your body reaches a state of ketosis, your brain receives and uses more ketones. These ketones have been scientifically proven to be responsible for controlling your ability to concentrate. In fact, lots of people who are in physically decent shape use the Keto diet to improve their mental performance. There is a common misconception that, for your brain to function properly, it requires a certain amount of carbohydrates. This gives some people the impression that, as the Keto diet is about limiting carbohydrate intake, it is may reduce your mental performance. This is not true.

After around 1-2 weeks of your brain adapting to the Keto diet, it uses the abundant supply of ketones that are increasing becoming available – this increases your mental performance. What tends to confuse people is that, before your brain adapts to this, you may suffer from side effects – symptoms of the Keto diet. This might be a headache, common cold, and difficulty concentrating. You must understand that, once your body has adapted and overcome this 'adaption' stage, you can enjoy the benefits that the Keto diet offers: higher energy levels, concentration, mood and overall mental health.

Improved Physical Endurance

As you progress further into the Keto diet, you might notice your physical endurance improve. There is a lot of scientific research to suggest that, as a Keto diet accesses all the energy stored in your fat reserves, it can significantly improve your physical endurance. Most people's bodies aren't using all this energy because not all their fat stores are available, especially if they eat a diet high in carbohydrates. Your body's ability to burn these carbohydrates (or glycogen) is limited to only a few hours when you're physically active, especially if you're working out. This might make you feel like eating before and after a workout, if you've been out walking, or even doing day to day chores like housekeeping. The keto diet solves this problem because, by restricting your carbohydrate intake, your body taps into energy stored in your fat reserves to feed your brain the vital ketones it needs.

A Treatment for Diabetes

Another benefit of the Keto diet is that it is a low carbohydrate diet. There is a lot of scientific research to suggest that the diet is an excellent remedy for controlling, or in some cases, even reversing type II diabetes. As you might know already, a high blood sugar level is a main factor in causing diabetes. For most people, the source of this sugar comes from the carbohydrates they eat. As the Keto diet is about limiting the carbohydrates you eat, it should be no surprise that the less of them you eat, the lower your blood sugar will be. This decrease in blood sugar is a natural benefit the Keto diet provides. However, as a word of caution, if you are a diabetic and want to start the Keto diet, you should speak to your doctor about your medications because you may have to adjust the amount you take to balance out this process.

THE SIDE EFFECTS OF
THE KETO DIET

CHAPTER 5

Keto Flu

Perhaps the most common side effect of the Keto diet, and one which I have personally experienced, is the Keto flu. When your body transitions to burning ketones, you may experience a few troublesome symptoms. The most common ones are: nausea, mood swings, muscle cramps and poor overall wellbeing. Personally speaking, nausea affected me the most when I made the transition. I know people who suffered a lot, and others who didn't suffer at all. What symptoms you have depends on your body and its ability to adapt to this change – don't worry though, as you will recover eventually!

There are a few things you can do to make this transition go more smoothly.

- **Gradually** reduce your carbohydrate intake. body is a machine and takes time to adjust. Allow time for the ketones to kick it. Create a meal plan that allows you to reduce your intake gradually over a few weeks to a month. In the meantime, drink a cup of bouillon to help alleviate these symptoms.

Bad Breath

This is probably going to be the most unwanted and embarrassing side effect for you. Bad breath is produced by acetone, which is a type of ketone your body produces during ketosis. It smells quite like bleach or cleaning fluid – an unpleasant smell you certainly don't want! Drinking alcohol can make this smell even worse too. Despite this, it is a positive thing because it tells you that your body is in a state of ketosis. I know people who suffered from bad breath a lot during the first few months, and others who didn't suffer at all. Whether you suffer from it depends on your body and its ability to adapt to this change – don't worry though, as you will recover eventually! Excellent oral hygiene is yet to preventing bad breath, so make sure you always carry around some dental spray, floss and gum.

DIETING PRINCIPLES

Before we introduce alcohol into the mix, let's recap what we have learnt so far. Here is a list of dieting principles that you must adhere to. They will help you achieve dieting success. They are as follows:

- Your daily calories should come from: carbohydrates 5% - 10%, fat 60% - 75% and protein 15% - 30%.
- You should not eat more than 50g of carbohydrates daily.
- You should try to eat monounsaturated fats, saturated fats and omega oils,
- You should not eat fruit and other snacks when you are close to your carb limit.
- You should not starve yourself – eat when you are hungry. Starving yourself long

term is a path to failure.

- You should always stick to reputable meal plans (see part III of this book).
- You should stock up non-starchy vegetables, eggs, avocado, meat and other fermented foods like tuna fish – you never know what disaster might prevent your next trip to the grocery store!
- You should not eat vegetable soils, hydrogenated oils, margarine, trans fat, soybean and corn oil.
- You should eat raw and organic dairy products like unpasteurized milk, not pasteurized milk.
- You should eat mushrooms, salmon, nuts and avocados to avoid an electrolyte deficiency.
- You should not eat processed foods. If you have no choice but to eat them, check out the nutritional labels to ensure you don't exceed your daily carbohydrate allowance.
- You should be wary of food packing that says 'fat-free' because these may contain hidden fats and salt.

- You should make sure to plan your diet one to two weeks in advance to avoid food and alcohol cravings (see part III: daily meal plan).

PART II
TO DRINK OR NOT TO DRINK?

HOW DOES MY BODY BURN ALCOHOL?

~CHAPTER 7~

Most of us are familiar with the three macronutrients, carbohydrate, fat, and protein, which make up most of our diets. Foods that fall into these categories are all processed by the body in similar ways. Carbohydrates, as we discussed, are the body's preferred source of fuel, and that's really all it is good for. Fat molecules are needed to facilitate some of the most important chemical reactions in the body, including making hormones.

Fat often gets the bad rap for weight gain. While it is true that a little bit of fat packs a big calorie punch, in moderation, fat can make you feel fuller, longer, and help you lose weight. Protein is primarily used for muscle growth and repair, and the amino acids that make it up are used to make neurotransmitters, the chemicals responsible for regulating our mood, among other things.

It seems that these three macronutrients have bodily functions covered, so where does alcohol fit in? Physiologically speaking, the answer is, nowhere. The body does not need alcohol, as evidenced by all of the people that completely abstain and live perfectly healthy lives. The body considers alcohol a toxin and does its best to eliminate it by burning it for energy and getting rid of the rest in urine. The liver can turn some of the alcohol into ketones that are burned for energy, but only if carbs are not available. The rest simply gets washed out, but not before causing damage to cells, especially those found in the liver.

The truth is that our bodies would probably be happy to never see another molecule of alcohol again, but that just isn't realistic for most people. Alcohol has been facilitating socialization for as long as history can remember. Recent studies have even shown the benefits of drinking certain alcohols, mainly wine, for decreasing stress and reducing the risk of heart disease. For the sake of this article, we will assume that a bit of light drinking is just fine.

Alcohol does affect the results of a Keto diet, however. Drinking pure alcohol, without any added sugars and mixers, will maintain ketosis. This is the good news. The bad news is, the ketones produced by processing alcohol will be burned for fuel instead of pulling fat from body stores for the same purpose. This means, if you consistently drink alcohol, your weight loss will be slowed, and may even come to a halt under certain conditions.

Dieting and maintaining ketosis can be difficult enough. We often socialize with food and drink, and limiting what you can eat to maintain ketosis can be a challenge. It would be nice to at least have a couple of cocktails to reconnect with friends. It is certainly possible to reach your weight loss goals through ketosis, and maintain a social life at the same time. You just need to learn how to do it right. The general guideline is to drink alcohol in moderation, just as with any other healthy eating plan.

Remember that alcohol is a toxin, and the less you consume, the better. Do your liver a favor and try to limit yourself to just a couple of drinks out with friends. Drinking less will speed your weight loss results, and make you feel better overall. Your body wastes energy trying to repair cells damaged by alcohol, leaving less energy for you to complete daily tasks, like exercising and working. We call this the hangover, something you may already be familiar

DRINKING ON THE KETO DIET

~CHAPTER 8~

This chapter may seem a little reminiscent of high school health class — but a much needed one at that! Truthfully, a drink here and there will not disrupt your diet plan, but over consuming regularly has its drawbacks. Deciding to try any weight loss plan, including the Keto diet requires a bit of a lifestyle change. Likely, you spent time out to dine, having a few cocktails with friends. Any time we decide to diet, we need to make some lifestyle changes to avoid falling back into unhealthy habits. Usually, this means cutting out alcohol, but there are ways to include some stress-relieving cocktails without derailing your social life altogether.

Did drinking cause you to gain weight in the first

place? Many people in their early twenties learn to binge-drink alcohol as a social norm. We go to college parties, stay out all night and have an enjoyable time. We end up drunk, spinning, and sick sometimes, making questionable decisions, to say the least. Not only are we over consuming calories through alcohol, but we are staying up later, and eating extra meals to 'soak up' the booze. Keep in mind that tactic doesn't reduce blood alcohol levels, it just reduces the effects.

Even if that isn't the case for you, remember that alcohol usually doesn't just mean alcohol. It also means excess calories and carbohydrates from added sugars. Indeed, you may have been drinking tequila, but the sugary margarita mix that went along with it loaded you with extra calories, quickly adding to your waistline. That margarita may seem refreshing and light, but just one 10-ounce drink can pack about 500 calories, comparable to a hearty dinner meal.

Pure alcohol, or ethanol, itself doesn't pose a threat to continuing ketosis, but we rarely drink anything without some sort of filler. We drink beers and wine, that pack extra carbohydrates and sugars. We mix hard liquor with juices and sickeningly-sweet mixers for effect, all of which are loaded with ketosis-killing sugars. This is what really gets us in trouble, whether on a standard calorie-restricted diet or with ketosis.

If you are used to sugary, novelty drinks out at the bar, it is time to reconsider your options. There are mixers that use artificial sweeteners, like sugar alcohols and aspartame, to replace sugar, but are not commonplace in the bar scene. Specific lines of drink boast the low-carb hype, but few fall within a reasonable restriction for a Keto diet. Remember that we are shooting for 10-15 grams of carbs per meal, and 50-60 grams per day. If you plan to eat as well, this leaves very little room for mixers of any kind.

The point of alcohol is to dull your senses and to impair your brain from making good choices. It is this effect that causes relaxation for most people, as stress usually has our minds whirling. We have all been there, where two drinks turn into three, and suddenly, you are drunk. There is a fine line between lightly buzzed and drunk, and it takes a bit of practice to know the difference. The general recommendation is to eat before you drink, as food, specifically carbohydrates, helps slow absorption of alcohol, delaying its effect on you. When you drink without eating, a beer or two may affect you much more than eating and having a couple. By this logic, the Keto diet may cause a problem.

The strict restriction of carbohydrates on the Keto diet means you will almost immediately feel the effects of alcohol, and you will have much less of a tolerance for it. For many, it may be hard to control just how many they have, so moderating and maintaining composure is a problem.

On the bright side, if you decide to partake in the festivities, one or two drinks may have you feeling good, without the need to drink anymore. You can effectively get a little buzz while consuming less alcohol, if you can stop yourself from having a third whilst out with friends. The fact that you are trying the Keto diet assumes that you care about your health and wellbeing. Over Consuming and damaging your liver and brain with alcohol does not jive with those goals. While a few nights here and there won't derail your fitness journey, but regular weekends of debauchery certainly will.

Studies show that regular consumption of alcohol inhibits certain vitamins and minerals from being absorbed in the body. The big ones are Thiamin, folic acid, and magnesium. Thiamin and all B vitamins are necessary for proper energy production, making you feel majorly sluggish with regular drinking. Folic acid is vital for cell regeneration. The body needs it to produce DNA and RNA, the building blocks of new cells. If you plan to become pregnant, a deficiency in folic acid can lead to birth defects. On that note, a Keto diet is generally not recommended during pregnancy because the baby needs carbohydrates to grow. Talk to your doctor if this is the case. Finally, magnesium is responsible for all sorts of things, but mainly for electrolyte balance. A common symptom of deficiency is leg cramps. It can also cause nausea, vomiting, and fatigue (classic hangover symptoms).

We can find these nutrients abundantly in foods, but lots of times, alcohol takes the place of food. People think they will not gain weight by skipping meals in favor of alcohol, but they are actually doing their bodies a major disservice by missing out on vital nutrients in the process If you are serious about getting your health in order, make sure to address the problem of overconsumption too. Cutting back will make you feel better, make you more productive and give you the general ability to handle life.

MAINTAINING KETOSIS WHILE DRINKING

Let's talk a little bit about how to safely incorporate alcohol into the Keto diet, now that I have scared you into never drinking again! Realistically, a few drinks here and there will not derail your goals, but consistent overindulgence can quickly thwart your best efforts. Having a solid plan of action before you head out for the night will help you navigate your way on the Keto diet while also maintaining your weight loss goals.

When you are first getting started with ketosis, a great idea is to abstain from alcohol for at least a couple of weeks while you adjust to the new diet. Besides having a much lower tolerance, drinking too much will keep your body from making its own ketones, slowing the process. Let your body get settled then consider adding in a cocktail or two.

First, we need to understand that the Keto diet is generally not a calorie-controlled diet, as that factor is largely weighed in by the available food choices. A strict diet of meat and vegetables has no other option but to be generally low-calorie, so watching calories on top of ketosis really isn't necessary. The general recommendation is to eat as much of the keto-friendly foods as you desire, provided, of course, you are within your carb limit.

More specifically, we need to consider the overall carbohydrate profile of our diet, including alcoholic drinks, as ketosis is all about maintaining that number. My best piece of advice is to do your research before heading to the bar and plan ahead. Think about what you will order ahead of time instead of just winging it. You may think that your vodka and club soda has no carbs, but that small splash of juice they added may just push you over the top. Think about what you want, and be very specific when you order.

Planning to ask the bartender about the carb content of anything behind the bar is a bad plan. They typically just know what goes into a drink, not the numbers. Anything in a bottle is unlikely to have the calorie and carb content listed on it unless it is marketed toward a diet-friendly consumer. If you have already met your carb goal for the day and can't live without a glass of wine as a nightcap, you risk slowing your weight loss progress by breaking ketosis. If you plan ahead, you can work that glass of wine into your dinner and suffer no consequences. As you develop your meal plan, have that glass of wine, or beverage of choice as an alternate option. In most cases, that will be like trading a higher-carb vegetable for a glass of wine.

Let's pretend for a moment that you are sitting at a bar. What on Earth are you supposed to order? Most people have a standard order, never fail, if no inspiration strikes them, they will order a Bud Light, or a Margarita, or whatever. Having done your research ahead of time, you find that both options may just be off the table. In certain situations, a Bud Light could do just fine, but only one.

Think about what we have learned so far: hard liquor has no added fillers that could contain carbs. Start the base of your drink with vodka, rum, gin, or whiskey. These are fine for ketosis, but brown liquors like whiskey and dark rum have more calories and have other substances that tend to make hangovers worse. The calories aren't terribly concerning. Make sure your liquor of choice is unflavored, or that whatever is added does not contain carbohydrates. Next, choose your mixer. There are so many options: pineapple juice, cranberry juice, cola, seltzer, the sky's the limit, just not if you are in ketosis. Most of these options have sugars, especially the juices and cola. Zero calorie seltzers and sodas are your best choice. If you are really into cranberry, a diet version has a couple grams of carbs, which could be worked into your plan.

If you are not used to drinking hard liquor and have not had a drink on ketosis, take it slow.

Alcohol tends to hit you much harder while following a Keto diet, and if you are used to drinking beer exclusively, that's a double negative. Have one drink, and wait awhile before trying another. Make sure someone is with you that can help if you start to get too tipsy. Even though your meal will be low-carb, eating anything before drinking will help your body digest it slower, making the onset of your buzz a little more normal.

BEER GUIDE

Beer is a wonderful, imbibing, bubbly glass of delicious. By this description, you may wonder if this writer is a little bias, and you would be right. The wonderful thing about beer is there are so many unusual flavors, types and ways to infuse assorted flavors. You could literally drink a different type of beer every single day and never run out of options.

Beer is made through the process of fermenting barley and hops. The idea is to extract the sugars found in these common grains, then ferment them using yeast to produce alcohol. These beverages range in alcohol content, but for the most part, a standard beer is about 5% alcohol, which is very light compared to hard liquor. Because of this fact, it is easy to have a beer after work, and still be able to drive home from the bar.

This fact is also the downfall of beer. Since it takes a bit more to get a buzz, we are subject to drinking more of the fine liquid, and all the carbs that come with it. Depending on the type of beer you are used to drinking, this could be a lot, or a lot, a lot. The problem with beer is that it comes from barley and hops, which are grains. Grains are full of sugars and carbs, making them non-existent in the standard Keto diet.

Dark beers typically have a higher concentration of these ingredients, or have added flavorings, like molasses, which is straight sugar. Beer can contain so many calories and carbohydrates that it is as filling as food to some people. Fun fact, during the Revolutionary War, soldiers were given rations of beer and whiskey in addition to food for calories, to take the edge off the prospect of war.

Light beers, like ales, have more of a chance of making it into a Keto diet but having more than a couple can quickly unravel your progress. Take a look at the following chart to see how your favorites stack up. You may need to suck it up and find alternatives to your go-to beers for now. On the bright side, you will meet your weight loss goals and possibly find a new favorite in the process.

The following table of beer options are all under 5 grams of carbohydrate but do vary in calories. The most important thing with the Keto diet is the carb content, however, and all of these options can reasonably fit alongside a low-carb mean plan.

Type of Beer	Calories	Carbs (grams)
Budweiser Select 55	55	1.8
Miller MGD 64	64	2.4
Budweiser Select	99	3.1
Anheuser-Busch Ice Lager	171	3.2
Beck's Premier Light	63	3.8
Amstel Light	95	5
Labatt Blue	153	5
Corona Light	99	5
Coors Light	102	5

You might notice that all the beers on this list are of a light, larger variety. Darker, fuller beers packing more flavor are darker because they are more concentrated with hops. While they may be your favorites, for the sake of your success on the Keto diet, you should aim to go with a lighter beer to stay within your carb limits.

WINE GUIDE

Just like beer, there are also plenty of options to choose from. Wine dates back centuries to early man. Imagine civilization thousands of years ago, sitting around talking about the new Egyptian pharaoh over a glass of red wine. The Egyptians were one of the first civilizations to begin fermenting grapes for wine, but not before Armenia, China and Greece.

There are two main types of wine: white and red. Under each type are multiple varieties, all of which have their droves of followers, and are distinguished by the grapes they are fermented from. With wine, the general rule of thumb is the dryer the better. In case you are not a wine connoisseur, dry wine means there is less sugar. The opposite, although not called wet, is very sweet. Your sweet rose or chardonnay is pretty much off limits for a Keto diet, but there are plenty of drier versions of wine to try. The table on the next page shows the popular types of wine and their carb count.

Type of wine	Carbs (grams, 4oz)
Zinfandel (red)	3.5
Cabernet Sauvignon (red)	3
Shiraz (red)	3
Pinot Noir (red)	2.7
Sauvignon blanc (white)	2.4
Pinot grigio (white)	2.4

You will notice that this list goes off a standard 4-ounce serving. This is equal to a half cup, or about half of a standard size wine glass (no big boy glasses here). If you are used to drinking larger quantities, a great tip to use with wine is cutting it with something fizzy. If you are not used to the flavor of dry wine, it may help to water it down with some seltzer water, either flavored or unflavored. Products do exist that do this for you, the standard wine cooler, but these are usually loaded with sugar to produce a specific taste. This can lead to an overwhelmingly sweet mixture with too many carbs to count. If you are looking to drink a few with friends while you socialize, having a total of one glass of wine over three glasses by cutting it can be a great way to give in to the oral fixation drinking gives you, but without the added calories and carbohydrates.

MIXED DRINKS GUIDE

The problem with mixed drinks is the mixer itself, not the alcohol. Any distilled, hard liquor is all alcohol, no carbohydrates unless there are flavors added. For example, whiskey with cinnamon flavor (like Fireball) is packed with sugar, about 10g per shot! Most of us don't drink these alcohols straight, as the concentrated alcohol is tough to take down. Instead, we make cocktails with these liquors with mixers that make them feel fancy.

Some of the most common mixers are juices, like orange or cranberry cocktail, or sodas like Sprite or Coca-Cola. While they make diet versions of most sodas and some juices, most bars just carry the standard stuff and cutting off the dieting crowds. Here and there, you may find a place that is enlightened to the idea of a low-carb drink, but you should bet on your own knowledge rather than the stock of the bar. It is possible to still have your favorite drinks, just modified to contain less sugar and fewer carbohydrates. The table on the next page shows you easy swaps for your favorite drinks.

Type of drink	Carbs (g)	Substitute	Carbs (g)
Rum and Coca-Cola	26	Coke Zero	0
Vodka Cran	18	Diet cranberry juice	2
-	-	Seltzer with cranberry	0.5
Arnold Palmer	22	Unsweetened tea Crystal light lemonade	0
Vodka Soda	20	Diet soda	0

Notice that using diet products and seltzers instead of heavy juices and sodas dramatically change the carb content of these drinks. Even if you were not on a carb-conscious diet, making these switches seems like a no brainer. Yes, these drinks still have calories, but adding the 20 grams of carbs in a vodka soda adds about 80 calories to the drink, just by choosing a full-sugar option. That hardly seems worth it!

THE TOP 10 ALCOHOLS FOR KETOSIS

Without any further ado, here is my list of top 10 alcohols you should drink on the keto diet. They are in order of carbohydrate content, and a variety of options for beer, wine, and mixed drinks are also included. Keep in mind that some of these options still contain minimal amounts of carbs, and that adds up quickly if you decide to have a few. Add them into your daily carb limit to enjoy the benefits of the keto diet while still maintaining an active social life.

1. John Daly (modified): 0 grams carbohydrate

   This drink is a refreshing mix of iced tea and lemonade. Most people think of

Arnold Palmer as the pioneer behind this mixture, but the addition of vodka makes it a John Daly. Naturally, most people make this with sweet tea and sugar-laden lemonade. However, it is still possible to enjoy the essence of this lovely drink by using mixer alternatives. Simply use unsweetened iced tea and Crystal Light lemonade to cut out the sugar. The lemonade is sweetened with artificial sweetener, so you won't be missing a thing! This drink is great as a summer favorite out on the patio.

2. Vodka and club soda: 0 grams carbohydrate.

This popular drink is great in a pinch. Every bar has diet soda and vodka, making this a versatile option even when pickings are slim. Add a bit of mint or a slice of lemon for a refreshing drink without the excess calories.

3. Rum and Coke Zero: 0 grams carbohydrate.

This popular refresher is great any time of year. The traditional Coca-Cola version is packed with excess sugar that could blow any diet. Make a simple swap for Diet Coke or Coke Zero for the same flavor without the guilt.

4. Budweiser Select 55: 1.8 g carbohydrate.

If beer is your thing, Budweiser has a low-carb option for you! Of all the beers out there, this variety is the best when it comes to the Keto diet. It is, of course, a light beer, so you stout lovers may not be totally impressed, but the familiar hops flavor will keep you coming back for more.

5. Vodka Cran: 2 grams carbohydrate.
Every bartender recognizes a Vodka Cran but they may use sweet cranberry juice cocktail for the mixture. Ask for Diet

Cranberry juice if it is available, or buy some to make at your next cocktail party at home.

6. Sauvignon blanc (white wine): 2.4g carbohydrate.

   If you're feeling fancy and light, this bubbly white wine will do just fine. With just a couple grams of carbohydrate, get your sophisticated flare on without the excess.

7. Pinot Grigio (white wine): 2.4 grams carbohydrate.

   Another wine favorite, Pinot Grigio is a popular white wine, found just about anywhere.

8. Miller MGD 64: 2.4 grams carbohydrate.

   This beer markets itself as the dieter's beer, and for good reason. With just 2.4 grams of carbohydrate, this could easily pair alongside a healthy grilled chicken salad out on the rooftop.

9. Cabernet Sauvignon (red wine): 3 grams carbohydrate.

If it's red wine you crave, this bold red is right up your alley. To enjoy it a little longer, try adding a bit of club soda to make it a sparkling sensation. You can have a big glass of the mixture without the excess carb.

10. Budweiser Select: 3.1 grams carbohydrate.

If you are looking for a fuller beer than the 55 or MGD 64, Bud Select will give that to you, but with a slight increase in carbs. You may simply feel it is worth it as the taste is much more interesting. Drink sparingly!

There you have it! My list of 10 perfectly viable drink options for the diehard Keto follower. Surely you will be able to find something on this list to enjoy, as you keep your social life in full swing. Next, let's take a look at Part 3 for some great tips on how to include these options into your meal plan.

PART III
MAINTAINING
PROGRESS

KEEPING UP THE HARD WORK

~CHAPTER 14~

Now we have established that you can easily make alcohol part of your life, let's talk about how to do it. Even though the drinks in this list don't contain large amounts of carbohydrates, they still have calories, and so they still count. Not to worry, as your tolerance for alcohol should drop dramatically when your body switches to burning ketones when you start the Keto diet, so drinking as much as you are used to might not be too likely. Anyhow, while the diet is not really focused on counting calories as such, having any alcoholic drink, and indeed food for that matter, in moderation is still a clever idea.

There are a lot of variables to consider when it comes to fitting alcohol in to your meal plan, or anything else that has a slightly higher carb content. The basis of the Keto diet is a strict carb restriction, so just about all your former favorite things will be off your shopping list just the same. To name a few, no bread, juice, pasta or rice. At this point, you have probably already determined that these things are off limits, so this should be no surprise. If you are still eating these kinds of things on a Keto meal plan, you are probably not in ketosis. If you are, please let us know what magic you have pulled out of your hat to make that work.

Now that the obvious is out of the way, we need to look at the rest of the diet. Unless a food is an animal protein or pure fat, like olive oil, it probably has carbohydrates. You are good with lean meats and oils, but vegetables and fruits have sugars, even if only minimal. Fruits are pretty much out of the question, as their natural sugars add up to a lot of carbohydrates. Just a handful of grapes has about 15 grams of carbs, your maximum for any one meal, and way too much for a snack. If you were to substitute your entire carb allotment for this handful of grapes, you will be hungry.

The trick to the Keto diet is to eat enough bulk through the fiber in addition to proteins and fats to make up for the lack of carbohydrates. For example, you could either have the half cup of grapes alongside some protein, or you could have a heaping plate of salad. Which do you think would satisfy you longer? Likely the salad, unless you really have a thing for grapes. Staying within your carb limits is completely possible, it just takes some planning.

Take a look at the table below for a list of low-carb vegetables. Remember that the goal is to reach 15 grams per meal, not to get as low as possible. Feel free to eat the veggies abundantly. You simply must stack them in your meals until you reach your limit, add a protein and you're done. Fats should still be used in moderation as they are high calorie in large quantities, but sprinkle them on as a condiment. For example, olive oil and avocado on a salad dressing. Feel free to cook with a little bit of oil as well.

Vegetable	Carbs (g)
Olives, 5	0.1g
Arugula (1/2 cup)	0.2g
Spinach	0.2g
Lettuce (1/2 cup)	0.5g
Turnip greens (1/2 cup)	0.5g
Artichoke (1 heart)	1g
Pickle (1 large dill)	1g
Avocado (1/4)	2g
Zucchini (1 c)	3g
Kale (1 cup)	4g
Green beans (1 cup)	4g
Broccoli (1 cup)	4g
Cauliflower (1 cup)	4g
Tomato (1/2 cup)	5g

DAILY MEAL PLAN

CHAPTER 15

Breakfast
Eggs with Keto Hash

There's nothing better than a nice big crispy hash for breakfast. It's my 'go to' food when I'm in a hurry and don't have the time to stand around making something more involved. The best thing about hash is that it's quick to make. I like mine with a nice big zucchini thrown in, but you can also use a range of vegetables– whatever takes your fancy! Be sure to top the hash with a fried egg too! Eggs are naturally carb-free, so feel free to load up. Aim your portion size for 15 grams carbs between vegetables.

Cooking time
20 – 25 minutes

Ingredients (4 Servings):

- One 200g (7.1oz) zucchini.
- Two 60g (2.1oz) slices of bacon.
- Half of a 30g (1.1oz) onion.
- 1 Tablespoon of coconut oil.
- 1 Tablespoon chopped chives.
- Quarter teaspoon of salt.
- 1 large egg.

How to Make

1. Peel the onion and chop it into fine pieces.
2. Slice the bacon into fine pieces.
3. Place the chopped onion into a frying pan and place on a medium heat.
4. Add the chopped bacon and stir until a golden brown.
5. Chop the zucchini into fine pieces, and throw it into the pan.
6. Cook for 10 minutes until a golden brown.
7. Scrap the Hash onto a plate and garnish with finely chopped parsley.
8. Top the Hash with a fried egg.

Nutritional Values	Quantity (g)
Carbohydrate	9.1
Fiber	2.5
Net Carbs	6.6
Protein	17.4
Fat	35.5
of which saturated	15.7
Energy	423 kcal

In terms of Keto Diet rules, this meal provides:

Carbs	6%
Protein	17%
Fat	77%

Snack
Fat Bombs

These little beauties are both nutritious and filling. There's nothing better than feeling that coconut melt in your mouth, especially on a frosty winter day. While you can use nut and seed butter when making the bombs, I find coconut and pecan tastier – it's a matter of personal preference as to which choice of butter you should use. They taste best when stored in the fridge, and can be eaten as a quick tasty source of energy.

Cooking time
20 minutes

Ingredients (6 Servings):

- One 250g (8.9 oz) cup of coconut butter
- One 40g (1.4oz) cup of powdered Erythritol
- One teaspoon of sugar free maple syrup
- One 100g (3.5oz) cup of vanilla powder.

- One 55g (1.9oz) cup of extra virgin coconut oil
- One teaspoon of cinnamon
- 100g (3.5oz) of dark chocolate
- 28g (1oz) of cocoa butter

How to Make

1. Mix the coconut butter together with the powdered Erythritol in a bowl.
2. Add the extra virgin coconut oil.
3. Add the maple syrup.
4. Add the cinnamon
5. Mix well.
6. Place into the fridge for 30 minutes.
7. Fill a medium sized saucepan with water.
8. Place the dark chocolate together with the cocoa butter in a glass bowl
9. Place the bowl over the saucepan.
10. Melt the chocolate.
11. Once melted, place to cool.
12. From this chocolate, use your hands to create 10 small bars.
13. Place these bars onto a tray lined with baking

paper.

14. Place in the fridge to cool for 30 minutes.
15. Take the bars out of the fridge, and drizzle the coconut mixture onto the bars.
16. Enjoy!

In terms of Keto Diet rules, this meal provides:

Carbs	5%
Protein	19%
Fat	76%

Nutritional Values	Quantity (g)
Carbohydrate	9.5
Fiber	5.1
Net Carbs	4.3
Protein	16
Fat	28.8
of which saturated	14.7
Energy	355 kcal

Dinner

Oven Baked Southern Fried Chicken

Whether you're wanting an easy dinner, picnic meal, or a lunchbox treat, oven baked southern fried chicken is your best friend! The mouthwatering juiciness of the butter brined chicken pieces, together with the zesty herbs and spices makes for a wonderful taste-bud tingling experience.

Cooking time
15 minutes

Ingredients (3 Servings):

- 6 chicken drumsticks (0.8kg or 1.75.lb)
- Two 470ml (16 oz) cups of unsweetened almond milk.
- 1 Tablespoons of lemon juice.
- 1 Tablespoons of sea salt.
- 1 Teaspoons of black pepper.
- 1 Teaspoons of dried oregano.

- 1 Teaspoons of paprika.
- 1/2 teaspoon of garlic powder.
- 1/2 teaspoon of onion powder.
- 1/2 cup pork rinds.
- 15g (0.6oz) coconut flou

How to Make

1. Pour the almond milk, together with the lemon juice, oregano, salt, and pepper into a bowl.
2. Mix for about 1 minute.
3. Place the chicken drumsticks into this mixture.
4. Leave the chicken to brine in the mixture for 2 hours.
5. Place the paprika, onion power, garlic powder, pork rinds and coconut flour into a food processor.
6. Mix until finely crumbed.
7. Pre-heat your oven to 350F (180 C).
8. Place the crumbed coating onto a tray.
9. Place the chicken pieces onto the tray and evenly coat them in crumbs.
10. Place the coated chicken onto a lined

baking tray.

11. Bake for 50 minutes

In terms of Keto Diet rules, this meal provides:

Carbs	3%
Protein	44%
Fat	53%

Nutritional Values	Quantity (g)
Carbohydrate	1.9
Fiber	0.85
Net Carbs	1
Protein	15.8
Fat	8.55
of which saturated	3.2
Energy	157 kcal

Drink
Delicious Low Carb Cocktail

This drink is low in carbs and tastes great! On my list of the top 10 alcohols to drink on the Keto diet, this drink ranks about 9th or 10th place. This is an excellent position considering that this is a cocktail. As such, it's more of a guilty pleasure, and shouldn't be a drink to consume regularly. Although there are very little carbs in this drink, you might remember in the earlier chapters reading about how your body doesn't store alcohol; it metabolizes it instead. If you drink too many of these drinks, your metabolism will burn the alcohol, not your body fat as intended – this will delay ketosis. Moderation is key!

Cooking time
5 minutes

Ingredients (1 Serving):

- 80ml (2.7 fl oz) of fresh lime juice.

- 120ml (4 fl oz) of gin.
- 2 cups of water.
- Ice cubes.
- Fresh mint.
- A slice of cucumber – if it takes your fancy!

How to Make

1. Put the mint leaves into an ice cube tray.
2. Fill the tray with water.
3. Place the tray into the freezer.
4. Cut a slice of cucumber.
5. Place a couple of ice cubes into a cocktail glass.
6. Pour the gin, together with the lime juice, into the glass.
7. Pour the water into the glass.
8. To finish, top the glass with the slice of cucumber.

In terms of Keto Diet rules, this drink provides:

Carbs	93%
Protein	5%
Fat	2%

Nutritional Values	Quantity (g)
Carbohydrate	3.4
Fiber	0.2
Net Carbs	3.2
Protein	0.2
Fat	0
of which saturated	0
Energy	139 kcal

While there are certainly more options to choose from, the basic framework of the plan will remain the same. You will need a carbohydrate, a protein and a fat at each meal. As for alcohol, always make sure you choose a beverage that balances well you're your daily carb limit. If your meal plan is lower in carbs, you may compensate by having a beverage like the low carb cocktail that has around 3.5g of carbs at most – striking a fine balance is key to your success.

FAQs

CHAPTER 16

Q: What is ketosis?

A: Ketosis occurs as an alternative method for your body to produce energy. Our metabolism prefers to run off sugars from dietary carbohydrates, as they are simple and quick to convert to usable energy. The body stores excess energy as fat, generally when we overeat. Ketosis is the body's backup plan for when dietary fuel is not available. It pulls fat from storage and converts it to energy. Ketones are the by-products.

Q: How do I know if I am in Ketosis?

A: Some people have physical signs that their metabolism is in transition, including flu-like symptoms like a headache and nausea. As the transition finishes, most report feeling much better, and the assumption is that ketosis has set in. Some people never have this reaction, so the only surefire way to tell is by testing your urine. Use ketone strips, found at your local pharmacy to monitor ketones.

Q: I would like to include alcohol in my diet plan. I can't live without a glass of wine with dinner!

A: You may want to consider abstaining from alcohol for a couple of weeks while your body transitions to ketosis, as alcohol keeps your body from making ketones out of fat. Once you have established your diet, including a glass of wine with dinner is as simple as adding it to your total carb (aim for 15 grams) for your meal.

Q: I am used to drinking protein shakes for breakfast. Can I still do that?

A: There is nothing inherently wrong with protein shakes, but they often do contain carbohydrates. Also, most people mix it with fruit juices and frozen berries, which are off limits on the keto diet. Find a shake variety that is low carb and drink it with water. You may have to compromise and choose this as a snack option, as many varieties offer too many carbs for the amount of protein in the shake. Settle for a smaller snack serving with less protein, and eat something more substantial for breakfast.

Q: Should I just eat more protein to avoid carbs?

A: This is a complicated answer because yes, you will likely be increasing the serving size of your protein a bit. However, overdoing it on protein can be tough on your stomach and your wallet. Since your metabolism will be happy burning fat, increasing healthy oils like olive and avocado is a fantastic way to get those calories in without overfilling your stomach!

Q: What happens if I overdo it with drinks and go above and beyond my carb restriction?

A: First off, remember that the 50-60-gram carb restriction is a recommendation that may not fit everyone perfectly. However, having a couple extra drinks and exceeding that number may or not throw you out of ketosis, depending on your metabolism. Doing this once and a while likely won't diminish your results too much, but it may take a day or two to get back to burning fat exclusively. More frequent carb overdoses will make it much harder to continue losing weight, as your body tries to figure out where its energy source is coming from.

Q: What about cheat days

A: Most dieters plan in so-called 'cheat-days' to enjoy some of the things they have been missing. Since the Keto diet is solely based on how many carbs you eat, having regular cheat days really isn't a clever idea. If you do try intermittent ketosis, an emerging trend, adding scheduled cheat days with a bit of control can work long term, but your potential weight loss could slow.

Q: What is ketoacidosis? Should I be concerned?

A: If you have researched the Keto diet, you have

likely come across this term. Ketoacidosis refers to a dangerous condition in which the body cannot burn carbohydrates for energy. This happens mostly in diabetics, who have a functional problem processing the sugar. Cells cannot absorb the sugar due to the lack of insulin. The result is ketones building up to dangerous levels in the body, causing a multitude of health problems. The major difference is that this occurs when carbohydrates are present in the diet. Under planned ketosis, ketones are burned for fuel, and the excess is flushed out, with no health issues.

Q: Is using artificial sweeteners in drinks instead of sugar safe?

A: Recent studies have called out artificial sweeteners, specifically aspartame, as being a possible carcinogen (causes cancer). If you are concerned about common drink mixers with aspartame, use natural options like club soda or a splash of juice for added flavor. In general, the Keto diet can be planned in a way those whole foods are used instead of artificial options, so an artificially sweetened drink here and there isn't much cause for concern.

KETO QUIZ

Test your knowledge with this quick quiz. Not to worry, you won't be graded, and the answers are on the next page (no peeking)!

What is the average daily carbohydrate recommendation to reach ketosis?

- 50-100 grams
- 50-60 grams
- 40-60 grams

What is the biggest concern with alcohol and ketosis?

- Added calories
- Carbohydrates
- Fat

How many MGD 64 could you drink with dinner if

you have 10 grams worth of vegetables already on your plate?

- 1
- 2

ANSWERS

What is the average daily carbohydrate recommendation to reach ketosis?

50-60 grams

What is the biggest concern with alcohol and ketosis?

Carbohydrates. Naturally in beer and wine, heavy in mixers used with hard liquor. Flavored hard liquors usually have added sugars as well.

How many MGD 64 could you drink with dinner if you have 10 grams worth of vegetables already on your plate?

2. the goal is 15 grams of carb per meal, each MGD64 is 2.4 grams, so having 2 will bring you to a total of 14.8 grams of carbohydrate for the meal.

CONCLUSION

Thank for making it through to the end of the name of The Keto Diet and Alcohol: To drink, or not to drink? The beginner's guide to the top 10 drinks for weight loss. I do hope this book was informative and able to provide you with all the tools you need to achieve your goals of losing weight with the Keto diet without sacrificing your social life.

Remember, your carb goal for the day is 50-60 grams. This breaks down to about 15 grams at each meal, breakfast, lunch, and dinner. Include one snack during the day with about 10 grams of carbohydrate – though this depends on how many carbs are in your other meals. Balance is key. You should make use of the tables in this book to look up the carb content of specific items. This will provide a starting point for your research.

Once you begin using the same ingredients

repeatedly, it will become second nature to you, but the key is to stay vigilant of carbs and alcoholic drinks to avoid falling out of ketosis. My ultimate advice is to get creative and keep your meal plan interesting. Try new vegetables and cook with new spices for new flavors. In general, spices are carb free, so feel free to load them on. You will find that salad is a go-to option for lunches and dinner. By using a variety of spices, your salad can look different every day. Taco seasoning makes taco salad, while Italian dressing gives a salad a whole other flavor. Using different proteins, like tuna, chicken, steak or eggs help add some changes as well. A sense of discovery is key to quashing those cravings!

You might notice that vegetarian proteins like tofu or edamame have not been mentioned, and that is for good reason. Legumes and plant sources of protein also contain carbohydrates. If you can fit these starchy proteins into your daily carb allowance, go right ahead, but you are better off with meat, as this will satisfy you much longer than a vegetarian option. If you aren't sick of your favorite salad yet, you will be, so have something in your back pocket for variety.

Ultimately, most people feel that the Keto diet is limiting, as carbohydrates are a major factor in the diet. If you look optimistically at this challenge, you will quickly realize that the opportunities are endless. However, stay vigilant of alcohol. The list of the top 10 low carb alcohols I have provided you with here is not a means to an end. If you intend on drinking alcohol with every meal, refer to this list, but also remember that there may be other low carb options out there that may be right for you. The key to choosing the right food and alcohol for you is to peruse your favorite recipe websites – they will certainly intrigue your taste buds!

Finally, if you found this book useful in any way, a **review** on Amazon is always appreciated! This will certainly help us out here in Santa Monica.

Yours Truly,
Eva La Rouge.

Made in the USA
Lexington, KY
21 April 2018